The Slow Cooker Cookbook for Men

Hearty, Easy Meals Cooked Low and Slow

By Kelsey Cooper

Sommario

Introduction 7

Slow Cooker Side Dish Recipes 9

Introduction

We know you are constantly seeking easier means to prepare your meals. We likewise know you are probably tired investing long hrs in the cooking area food preparation with many frying pans and pots.

Well, now your search mores than! We found the excellent cooking area tool you can use from now on! We are discussing the Slow cooker! These fantastic pots permit you to prepare some of the most effective meals ever before with minimum initiative Slow cookers prepare your dishes easier and also a whole lot healthier! You don't require to be an expert in the kitchen area to prepare several of one of the most scrumptious, flavorful, distinctive as well as rich dishes! All you need is your Slow cooker as well as the ideal components! It will show you that you can make some remarkable morning meals, lunch recipes, side recipes, poultry, meat as well as fish recipes.

Finally yet significantly, this recipe book offers you some easy and sweet treats.

Barley Mix

Preparation time: 10 minutes

Cooking time: 6 hours

Servings: 2

Ingredients:

- 1 red onion, sliced

- ½ teaspoon sweet paprika

- ½ teaspoon turmeric powder

- 1 cup barley

- 1 cup veggie stock

- A pinch of salt and black pepper

- 1 garlic clove, minced

Directions:

1. In your slow cooker, mix the barley with the onion, paprika and the other ingredients, toss, put the lid on and cook on Low for 6 hours.

2. Divide between plates and serve as a side dish.

Nutrition: calories 160, fat 3, fiber 7, carbs 13, protein 7

Sweet Potato Mash

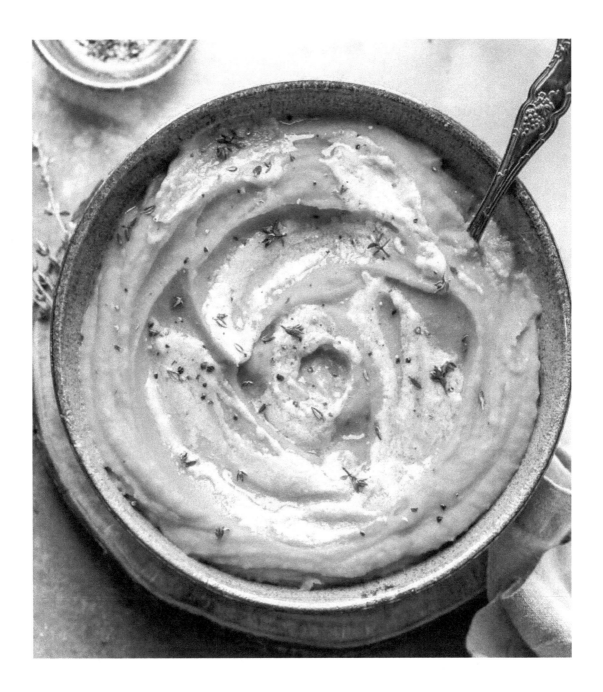

Preparation time: 10 minutes

Cooking time: 5 hours

Servings: 6

Ingredients:

- 2 pounds sweet potatoes, peeled and sliced

- 1 tablespoon cinnamon powder

- 1 cup apple juice

- 1 teaspoon nutmeg, ground

- ¼ teaspoon cloves, ground

- ½ teaspoon allspice

- 1 tablespoon butter, melted

Directions:

1. In your Slow cooker, mix sweet potatoes with cinnamon, apple juice, nutmeg, cloves and allspice, stir, cover and cook on Low for 5 hours.

2. Mash using a potato masher, add butter, whisk well, divide between plates and serve as a side dish.

Nutrition: calories 111, fat 2, fiber 2, carbs 16, protein 3

Lime Beans Mix

Preparation time: 10 minutes

Cooking time: 8 hours

Servings: 2

Ingredients:

- ½ pound lima beans, soaked for 6 hours and drained

- 1 tablespoon olive oil

- 2 scallions, chopped

- 1 carrot, chopped

- 2 tablespoons tomato paste

- 1 garlic cloves, minced

- A pinch of salt and black pepper to the taste

- 3 cups water

- A pinch of red pepper, crushed

- 2 tablespoons parsley, chopped

Directions:

1. In your slow cooker, mix the beans with the scallions, oil and the other ingredients, toss, put the lid on and cook on Low for 8 hours.

2. Divide between plates and serve as a side dish/

Nutrition: calories 160, fat 3, fiber 7, carbs 9, protein 12

Dill Cauliflower Mash

Preparation time: 10 minutes

Cooking time: 5 hours

Servings: 6

Ingredients:

- 1 cauliflower head, florets separated

- 1/3 cup dill, chopped

- 6 garlic cloves

- 2 tablespoons butter, melted

- A pinch of salt and black pepper

Directions:

1. Put cauliflower in your Slow cooker, add dill, garlic and water to cover cauliflower, cover and cook on High for 5 hours.

2. Drain cauliflower and dill, add salt, pepper and butter, mash using a potato masher, whisk well and serve as a side dish.

Nutrition: calories 187, fat 4, fiber 5, carbs 12, protein 3

Creamy Beans

Preparation time: 10 minutes

Cooking time: 2 hours

Servings: 2

Ingredients:

- 2 ounces green beans, trimmed and halved

- 2 tablespoons hot sauce

- 2 tablespoons heavy cream

- ½ cup coconut milk

- ¼ teaspoon cumin, ground

- ¼ tablespoon chili powder

Directions:

1. In your slow cooker, mix the beans with the hot sauce and the other ingredients, toss, put the lid on and cook on Low for 2 hours.

2. Divide between plates and serve right away as a side dish.

Nutrition: calories 230, fat 4, fiber 6, carbs 8, protein 10

Eggplant and Kale Mix

Preparation time: 10 minutes

Cooking time: 2 hours

Servings: 6

Ingredients:

- 14 ounces canned roasted tomatoes and garlic

- 4 cups eggplant, cubed

- 1 yellow bell pepper, chopped

- 1 red onion, cut into medium wedges

- 4 cups kale leaves

- 2 tablespoons olive oil

- 1 teaspoon mustard

- 3 tablespoons red vinegar

- 1 garlic clove, minced

- Salt and black pepper to the taste

- ½ cup basil, chopped

Directions:

1. In your Slow cooker, mix the eggplant with tomatoes, bell pepper and onion, toss, cover and cook on High for 2 hours.

2. Add kale, toss, cover slow cooker and leave aside for now.

3. In a bowl, mix oil with vinegar, mustard, garlic, salt and pepper and whisk well.

4. Add this over eggplant mix, also add basil, toss, divide between plates and serve as a side dish.

Nutrition: calories 251, fat 9, fiber 6, carbs 34, protein 8

Spinach Mix

Preparation time: 10 minutes

Cooking time: 1 hour

Servings: 2

Ingredients:

- 1 pound baby spinach

- ½ cup cherry tomatoes, halved

- ½ tablespoon olive oil

- ½ cup veggie stock

- 1 small yellow onion, chopped

- ¼ teaspoon coriander, ground

- ¼ teaspoon cumin, ground

- ¼ teaspoon garam masala

- ¼ teaspoon chili powder

- Salt and black pepper to the taste

Directions:

1. In your slow cooker, mix the spinach with the tomatoes, oil and the other ingredients, toss, put the lid on and cook on High for 1 hour.

2. Divide between plates and serve as a side dish.,

Nutrition: calories 270, fat 4, fiber 6, carbs 8, protein 12

Thai Side Salad

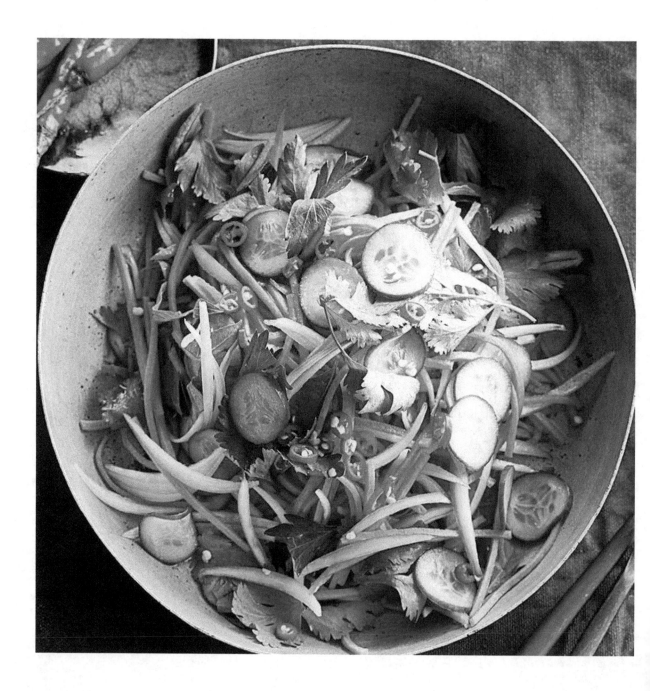

Preparation time: 10 minutes

Cooking time: 3 hours

Servings: 8

Ingredients:

- 8 ounces yellow summer squash, peeled and roughly chopped

- 12 ounces zucchini, halved and sliced

- 2 cups button mushrooms, quartered

- 1 red sweet potatoes, chopped

- 2 leeks, sliced

- 2 tablespoons veggie stock

- 2 garlic cloves, minced

- 2 tablespoon Thai red curry paste

- 1 tablespoon ginger, grated

- 1/3 cup coconut milk

- ¼ cup basil, chopped

Directions:

3. In your Slow cooker, mix zucchini with summer squash, mushrooms, red pepper, leeks, garlic, stock, curry paste, ginger, coconut milk and basil, toss, cover and cook on Low for 3 hours.

4. Stir your Thai mix one more time, divide between plates and serve as a side dish.

Nutrition: calories 69, fat 2, fiber 2, carbs 8, protein 2

Bbq Beans

Preparation time: 10 minutes

Cooking time: 8 hours

Servings: 2

Ingredients:

- ¼ pound navy beans, soaked overnight and drained

- 1 cup bbq sauce

- 1 tablespoon sugar

- 1 tablespoon ketchup

- 1 tablespoon water

- 1 tablespoon apple cider vinegar

- 1 tablespoon olive oil

- 1 tablespoon soy sauce

Directions:

1. In your slow cooker, mix the beans with the sauce, sugar and the other ingredients, toss, put the lid on and cook on Low for 8 hours.

2. Divide between plates and serve as a side dish.

Nutrition: calories 430, fat 7, fiber 8, carbs 15, protein 19

Rosemary Potatoes

Preparation time: 10 minutes

Cooking time: 3 hours

Servings: 12

Ingredients:

- 2 tablespoons olive oil

- 3 pounds new potatoes, halved

- 7 garlic cloves, minced

- 1 tablespoon rosemary, chopped

- A pinch of salt and black pepper

Directions:

2. In your Slow cooker, mix oil with potatoes, garlic, rosemary, salt and pepper, toss, cover and cook on High for 3 hours.

3. Divide between plates and serve as a side dish.

Nutrition: calories 102, fat 2, fiber 2, carbs 18, protein 2

White Beans Mix

Preparation time: 10 minutes

Cooking time: 6 hours

Servings: 4

Ingredients:

- 1 celery stalk, chopped

- 2 garlic cloves, minced

- 1 carrot, chopped

- 1 cup veggie stock

- ½ cup canned tomatoes, crushed

- ½ teaspoon chili powder

- ½ tablespoon Italian seasoning

- 15 ounces canned white beans, drained

- 1 tablespoon parsley, chopped

Directions:

1. In your slow cooker, mix the beans with the celery, garlic and the other ingredients, toss, put the lid on and cook on Low for 6 hours.

2. Divide the mix between plates and serve.

Nutrition: calories 223, fat 3, fiber 7, carbs 10, protein 7

Maple Brussels Sprouts

Preparation time: 10 minutes

Cooking time: 3 hours

Servings: 12

Ingredients:

- 1 cup red onion, chopped

- 2 pounds Brussels sprouts, trimmed and halved

- Salt and black pepper to the taste

- ¼ cup apple juice

- 3 tablespoons olive oil

- ¼ cup maple syrup

- 1 tablespoon thyme, chopped

Directions:

3. In your slow cooker, mix Brussels sprouts with onion, salt, pepper and apple juice, toss, cover and cook on Low for 3 hours.

4. In a bowl, mix maple syrup with oil and thyme, whisk really well, add over Brussels sprouts, toss well, divide between plates and serve as a side dish.

Nutrition: calories 100, fat 4, fiber 4, carbs 14, protein 3

Sweet Potato and Cauliflower Mix

Preparation time: 10 minutes

Cooking time: 4 hours

Servings: 2

Ingredients:

- 2 sweet potatoes, peeled and cubed

- 1 cup cauliflower florets

- ½ cup coconut milk

- 1 teaspoons sriracha sauce

- A pinch of salt and black pepper

- ½ tablespoon sugar

- 1 tablespoon red curry paste

- 3 ounces white mushrooms, roughly chopped

- 2 tablespoons cilantro, chopped

Directions:

1. In your slow cooker, mix the sweet potatoes with the cauliflower and the other ingredients, toss, put the lid on and cook on Low for 4 hours.

2. Divide between plates and serve as a side dish.

Nutrition: calories 200, fat 3, fiber 5, carbs 15, protein 12

Beets and Carrots

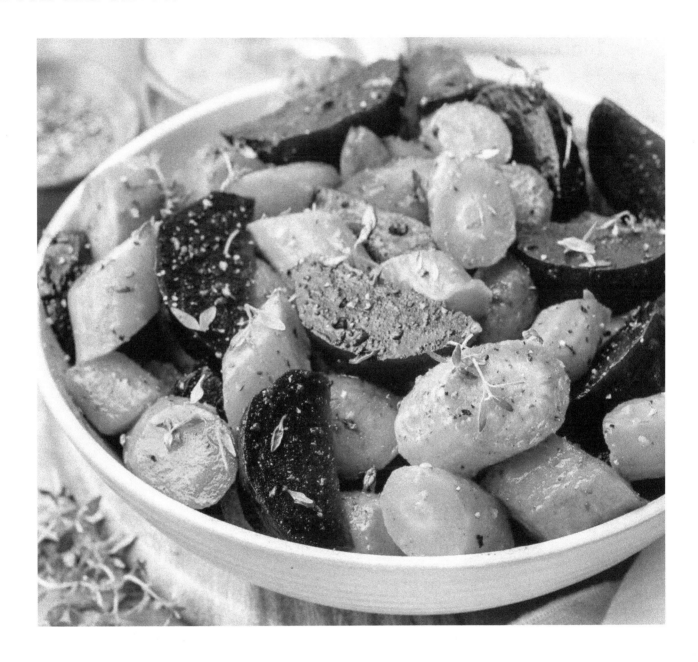

Preparation time: 10 minutes

Cooking time: 7 hours

Servings: 8

Ingredients:

- 2 tablespoons stevia

- ¾ cup pomegranate juice

- 2 teaspoons ginger, grated

- 2 and ½ pounds beets, peeled and cut into wedges

- 12 ounces carrots, cut into medium wedges

Directions:

1. In your Slow cooker, mix beets with carrots, ginger, stevia and pomegranate juice, toss, cover and cook on Low for 7 hours.

2. Divide between plates and serve as a side dish.

Nutrition: calories 125, fat 0, fiber 4, carbs 28, protein 3

Cabbage Mix

Preparation time: 10 minutes

Cooking time: 6 hours

Servings: 2

Ingredients:

- 1 pound red cabbage, shredded

- 1 apple, peeled, cored and roughly chopped

- A pinch of salt and black pepper to the taste

- ¼ cup chicken stock

- 1 tablespoon mustard

- ½ tablespoon olive oil

Directions:

1. In your slow cooker, mix the cabbage with the apple and the other ingredients, toss, put the lid on and cook on Low for 6 hours.

2. Divide between plates and serve as a side dish.

Nutrition: calories 200, fat 4, fiber 2, carbs 8, protein 6

Italian Veggie Mix

Preparation time: 10 minutes

Cooking time: 6 hours

Servings: 8

Ingredients:

- 38 ounces canned cannellini beans, drained

- 1 yellow onion, chopped

- ¼ cup basil pesto

- 19 ounces canned fava beans, drained

- 4 garlic cloves, minced

- 1 and ½ teaspoon Italian seasoning, dried and crushed

- 1 tomato, chopped

- 15 ounces already cooked polenta, cut into medium pieces

- 2 cups spinach

- 1 cup radicchio, torn

Directions:

1. In your Slow cooker, mix cannellini beans with fava beans, basil pesto, onion, garlic, Italian seasoning, polenta, tomato, spinach and radicchio, toss, cover and cook on Low for 6 hours.

2. Divide between plates and serve as a side dish.

Nutrition: calories 364, fat 12, fiber 10, carbs 45, protein 21

Parsley Mushroom Mix

Preparation time: 10 minutes

Cooking time: 4 hours

Servings: 2

Ingredients:

- 1 pound brown mushrooms, halved

- 2 garlic cloves, minced

- A pinch of basil, dried

- A pinch of oregano, dried

- ½ cup veggie stock

- Salt and black pepper to the taste

- 1 tablespoon olive oil

- 1 tablespoon parsley, chopped

Directions:

1. In your slow cooker, mix the mushrooms with the garlic, basil and the other ingredients, toss, put the lid on and cook on Low for 4 hours.

2. Divide everything between plates and serve.

Nutrition: calories 122, fat 6, fiber 1, carbs 8, protein 5

Wild Rice and Barley Pilaf

Preparation time: 10 minutes

Cooking time: 7 hours

Servings: 12

Ingredients:

- ½ cup wild rice

- ½ cup barley

- 2/3 cup wheat berries

- 27 ounces veggie stock

- 2 cups baby lima beans

- 1 red bell pepper, chopped

- 1 yellow onion, chopped

- 1 tablespoon olive oil

- A pinch of salt and black pepper

- 1 teaspoon sage, dried and crushed

- 4 garlic cloves, minced

Directions:

1. In your Slow cooker, mix rice with barley, wheat berries, lima beans, bell pepper, onion, oil, salt, pepper, sage and garlic, stir, cover and cook on Low for 7 hours.

2. Stir one more time, divide between plates and serve as a side dish.

Nutrition: calories 168, fat 5, fiber 4, carbs 25, protein 6

Cinnamon Squash

Preparation time: 10 minutes

Cooking time: 4 hours

Servings: 2

Ingredients:

- 1 acorn squash, peeled and cut into medium wedges

- 1 cup coconut cream

- A pinch of cinnamon powder

- A pinch of salt and black pepper

Directions:

1. In your slow cooker, mix the squash with the cream and the other ingredients, toss, put the lid on and cook on Low for 4 hours.

2. Divide between plates and serve as a side dish.

Nutrition: calories 230, fat 3, fiber 3, carbs 10, protein 2

Apples and Potatoes

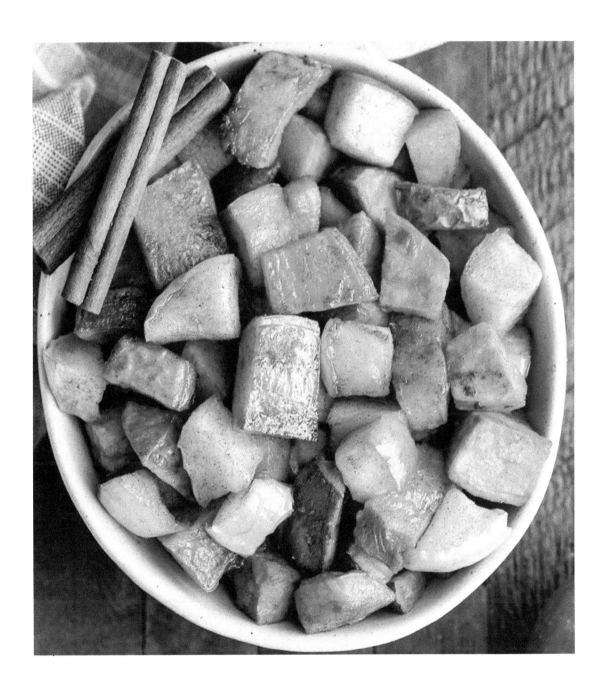

Preparation time: 10 minutes

Cooking time: 7 hours

Servings: 10

Ingredients:

- 2 green apples, cored and cut into wedges

- 3 pounds sweet potatoes, peeled and cut into medium wedges

- 1 cup coconut cream

- ½ cup dried cherries

- 1 cup apple butter

- 1 and ½ teaspoon pumpkin pie spice

Directions:

3. In your Slow cooker, mix sweet potatoes with green apples, cream, cherries, apple butter and spice, toss, cover and cook on Low for 7 hours.

4. Toss, divide between plates and serve as a side dish.

Nutrition: calories 351, fat 8, fiber 5, carbs 48, protein 2

Zucchini Mix

Preparation time: 10 minutes

Cooking time: 6 hours

Servings: 2

Ingredients:

- 1 pound zucchinis, sliced

- ½ teaspoon Italian seasoning

- ½ teaspoon sweet paprika

- Salt and black pepper

- ½ cup heavy cream

- ½ teaspoon garlic powder

- 1 tablespoon olive oil

Directions:

1. In your slow cooker, mix the zucchinis with the seasoning, paprika and the other ingredients, toss, put the lid on and cook on Low for 6 hours.

2. Divide between plates and serve as a side dish.

Nutrition: calories 170, fat 2, fiber 4, carbs 8, protein 5

Asparagus and Mushroom Mix

Preparation time: 10 minutes

Cooking time: 5 hours

Servings: 4

Ingredients:

- 2 pounds asparagus spears, cut into medium pieces

- 1 cup mushrooms, sliced

- A drizzle of olive oil

- Salt and black pepper to the taste

- 2 cups coconut milk

- 1 teaspoon Worcestershire sauce

- 5 eggs, whisked

Directions:

1. Grease your Slow cooker with the oil and spread asparagus and mushrooms on the bottom.

2. In a bowl, mix the eggs with milk, salt, pepper and Worcestershire sauce, whisk, pour into the slow cooker, toss everything, cover and cook on Low for 6 hours.

3. Divide between plates and serve as a side dish.

Nutrition: calories 211, fat 4, fiber 4, carbs 6, protein 5

Kale Mix

Preparation time: 10 minutes

Cooking time: 2 hours

Servings: 2

Ingredients:

- 1 pound baby kale

- ½ tablespoon tomato paste

- ½ cup chicken stock

- ½ teaspoon chili powder

- A pinch of salt and black pepper

- 1 tablespoon olive oil

- 1 small yellow onion, chopped

- 1 tablespoon apple cider vinegar

Directions:

5. In your slow cooker, mix the kale with the tomato paste, stock and the other ingredients, toss, put the lid on and cook on Low for 2 hours.

6. Divide between plates and serve as a side dish.

Nutrition: calories 200, fat 4, fiber 7, carbs 10, protein 3

Asparagus Mix

Preparation time: 10 minutes

Cooking time: 6 hours

Servings: 4

Ingredients:

- 10 ounces cream of celery

- 12 ounces asparagus, chopped

- 2 eggs, hard-boiled, peeled and sliced

- 1 cup cheddar cheese, shredded

- 1 teaspoon olive oil

Directions:

3. Grease your Slow cooker with the oil, add cream of celery and cheese to the slow cooker and stir.

4. Add asparagus and eggs, cover and cook on Low for 6 hours.

5. Divide between plates and serve as a side dish.

Nutrition: calories 241, fat 5, fiber 4, carbs 5, protein 12

Buttery Spinach

Preparation time: 10 minutes

Cooking time: 2 hours

Servings: 2

Ingredients:

- 1 pound baby spinach

- 1 cup heavy cream

- ½ teaspoon turmeric powder

- A pinch of salt and black pepper

- ½ teaspoon garam masala

- 2 tablespoons butter, melted

Directions:

1. In your slow cooker, mix the spinach with the cream and the other ingredients, toss, put the lid on and cook on Low for 2 hours.

2. Divide between plates and serve as a side dish.

Nutrition: calories 230, fat 12, fiber 2, carbs 9, protein 12

Chorizo and Cauliflower Mix

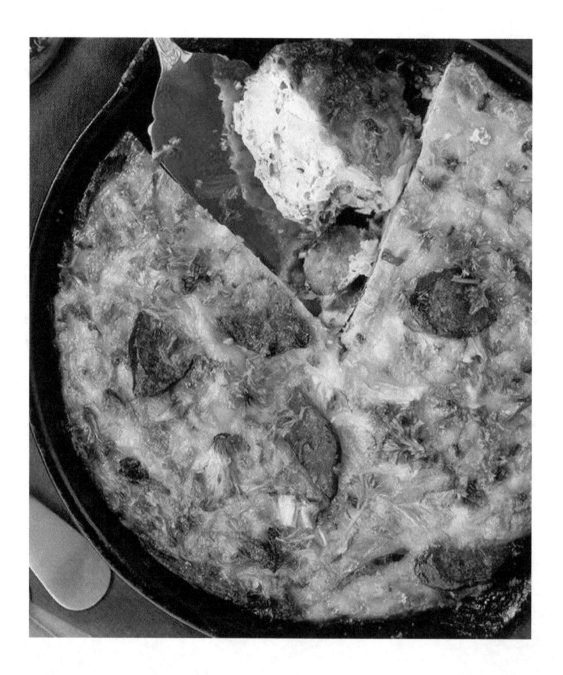

Preparation time: 10 minutes

Cooking time: 5 hours

Servings: 4

Ingredients:

- 1 pound chorizo, chopped

- 12 ounces canned green chilies, chopped

- 1 yellow onion, chopped

- ½ teaspoon garlic powder

- Salt and black pepper to the taste

- 1 cauliflower head, riced

- 2 tablespoons green onions, chopped

Directions:

1. Heat up a pan over medium heat, add chorizo and onion, stir, brown for a few minutes and transfer to your Slow cooker.

2. Add chilies, garlic powder, salt, pepper, cauliflower and green onions, toss, cover and cook on Low for 5 hours.

3. Divide between plates and serve as a side dish.

Nutrition: calories 350, fat 12, fiber 4, carbs 6, protein 20

Bacon Potatoes Mix

Preparation time: 10 minutes

Cooking time: 6 hours

Servings: 2

Ingredients:

- 2 sweet potatoes, peeled and cut into wedges

- 1 tablespoon balsamic vinegar

- ½ tablespoon sugar

- A pinch of salt and black pepper

- ¼ teaspoon sage, dried

- A pinch of thyme, dried

- 1 tablespoon olive oil

- ½ cup veggie stock

- 2 bacon slices, cooked and crumbled

Directions:

1. In your slow cooker, mix the potatoes with the vinegar, sugar and the other ingredients, toss, put the lid on and cook on Low for 6 hours

2. Divide between plates and serve as a side dish.

Nutrition: calories 209, fat 4, fiber 4, carbs 29, protein 4

Classic Veggies Mix

Preparation time: 10 minutes

Cooking time: 3 hours

Servings: 4

Ingredients:

- 1 and ½ cups red onion, cut into medium chunks

- 1 cup cherry tomatoes, halved

- 2 and ½ cups zucchini, sliced

- 2 cups yellow bell pepper, chopped

- 1 cup mushrooms, sliced

- 2 tablespoons basil, chopped

- 1 tablespoon thyme, chopped

- ½ cup olive oil

- ½ cup balsamic vinegar

Directions:

1. In your Slow cooker, mix onion pieces with tomatoes, zucchini, bell pepper, mushrooms, basil, thyme, oil and vinegar, toss to coat everything, cover and cook on High for 3 hours.

2. Divide between plates and serve as a side dish.

Nutrition: calories 150, fat 2, fiber 2, carbs 6, protein 5

Cauliflower Mash

Preparation time: 10 minutes

Cooking time: 5 hours

Servings: 2

Ingredients:

- 1 pound cauliflower florets

- ½ cup heavy cream

- 1 tablespoon dill, chopped

- 2 garlic cloves, minced

- 1 tablespoons butter, melted

- A pinch of salt and black pepper

Directions:

3. In your slow cooker, mix the cauliflower with the cream and the other ingredients, toss, put the lid on and cook on High for 5 hours.

4. Mash the mix, whisk, divide between plates and serve.

Nutrition: calories 187, fat 4, fiber 5, carbs 7, protein 3

Okra Side Dish

Preparation time: 10 minutes

Cooking time: 3 hours

Servings: 4

Ingredients:

- 2 cups okra, sliced

- 1 and ½ cups red onion, roughly chopped

- 1 cup cherry tomatoes, halved

- 2 and ½ cups zucchini, sliced

- 2 cups red and yellow bell peppers, sliced

- 1 cup white mushrooms, sliced

- ½ cup olive oil

- ½ cup balsamic vinegar

- 2 tablespoons basil, chopped

- 1 tablespoon thyme, chopped

Directions:

1. In your Slow cooker, mix okra with onion, tomatoes, zucchini, bell peppers, mushrooms, basil and thyme.

2. In a bowl mix oil with vinegar, whisk well, add to the slow cooker, cover and cook on High for 3 hours.

3. Divide between plates and serve as a side dish.

Nutrition: calories 233, fat 12, fiber 4, carbs 8, protein 4

Veggie Mix

Preparation time: 10 minutes

Cooking time: 5 hours

Servings: 2

Ingredients:

- 1 eggplant, cubed

- 1 cup cherry tomatoes, halved

- 1 small zucchini, halved and sliced

- ½ red bell pepper, chopped

- ½ cup tomato sauce

- 1 carrot, peeled and cubed

- 1 sweet potato, peeled and cubed

- A pinch of red pepper flakes, crushed

- 1 tablespoon basil, chopped

- 1 tablespoon parsley, chopped

- A pinch of salt and black pepper

- ½ cup veggie stock

- 1 tablespoon capers

- 1 tablespoon red wine vinegar

Directions:

1. In your slow cooker, mix the eggplant with the tomatoes, zucchini and the other ingredients, toss, put the lid on and cook on Low for 5 hours.

2. Divide between plates and serve as a side dish.

Nutrition: calories 100, fat 1, fiber 2, carbs 7, protein 5

Okra Side Dish

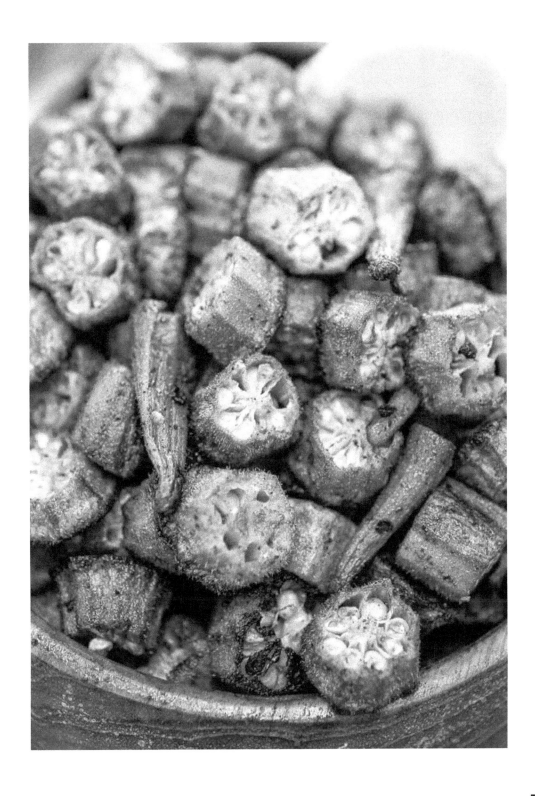

Preparation time: 10 minutes

Cooking time: 4 hours

Servings: 4

Ingredients:

- 1 pound okra, sliced

- 1 tomato, chopped

- 6 ounces tomato sauce

- 1 cup water

- Salt and black pepper to the taste

- 1 yellow onion, chopped

- 2 garlic cloves, minced

Directions:

1. In your Slow cooker, mix okra with tomato, tomato sauce, water, salt, pepper, onion and garlic, stir, cover and cook on Low for 4 hours.

2. Divide between plates and serve as a side dish.

Nutrition: calories 211, fat 4, fiber 6, carbs 17, protein 3

Farro Mix

Preparation time: 10 minutes

Cooking time: 4 hours

Servings: 2

Ingredients:

- 2 scallions, chopped

- 2 garlic cloves, minced

- 1 tablespoon olive oil

- 1 cup whole grain farro

- 2 cups chicken stock

- Salt and black pepper to the taste

- ½ tablespoon parsley, chopped

- 1 tablespoon cherries, dried

Directions:

1. In your slow cooker, mix the farro with the scallions, garlic and the other ingredients, toss, put the lid on and cook on Low for 4 hours.

2. Divide between plates and serve as a side dish.

Nutrition: calories 152, fat 4, fiber 5, carbs 20, protein 4

Okra Mix

Preparation time: 10 minutes

Cooking time: 8 hours

Servings: 4

Ingredients:

- 2 garlic cloves, minced

- 1 yellow onion, chopped

- 14 ounces tomato sauce

- 1 teaspoon sweet paprika

- 2 cups okra, sliced

- Salt and black pepper to the taste

Directions:

1. In your Slow cooker, mix garlic with the onion, tomato sauce, paprika, okra, salt and pepper, cover and cook on Low for 8 hours.

2. Divide between plates and serve as a side dish.

Nutrition: calories 200, fat 6, fiber 5, carbs 10, protein 4

Cumin Quinoa Pilaf

Preparation time: 10 minutes

Cooking time: 2 hours

Servings: 2

Ingredients:

- 1 cup quinoa

- 2 teaspoons butter, melted

- Salt and black pepper to the taste

- 1 teaspoon turmeric powder

- 2 cups chicken stock

- 1 teaspoon cumin, ground

Directions:

1. Grease your slow cooker with the butter, add the quinoa and the other ingredients, toss, put the lid on and cook on High for 2 hours

2. Divide between plates and serve as a side dish.

Nutrition: calories 152, fat 3, fiber 6, carbs 8, protein 4

Stewed Okra

Preparation time: 10 minutes

Cooking time: 3 hours

Servings: 4

Ingredients:

- 2 cups okra, sliced

- 2 garlic cloves, minced

- 6 ounces tomato sauce

- 1 red onion, chopped

- A pinch of cayenne peppers

- 1 teaspoon liquid smoke

- Salt and black pepper to the taste

Directions:

1. In your Slow cooker, mix okra with garlic, onion, cayenne, tomato sauce, liquid smoke, salt and pepper, cover, cook on Low for 3 hours.

2. Divide between plates and serve as a side dish.

Nutrition: calories 182, fat 3, fiber 6, carbs 8, protein 3

Saffron Risotto

Preparation time: 10 minutes

Cooking time: 2 hours

Servings: 2

Ingredients:

- ½ tablespoon olive oil

- ¼ teaspoon saffron powder

- 1 cup Arborio rice

- 2 cups veggie stock

- A pinch of salt and black pepper

- A pinch of cinnamon powder

- 1 tablespoon almonds, chopped

Directions:

1. In your slow cooker, mix the rice with the stock and the other ingredients, toss, put the lid on and cook on High for 2 hours.

2. Divide between plates and serve as a side dish.

Nutrition: calories 251, fat 4, fiber 7, carbs 29, protein 4

Okra and Corn

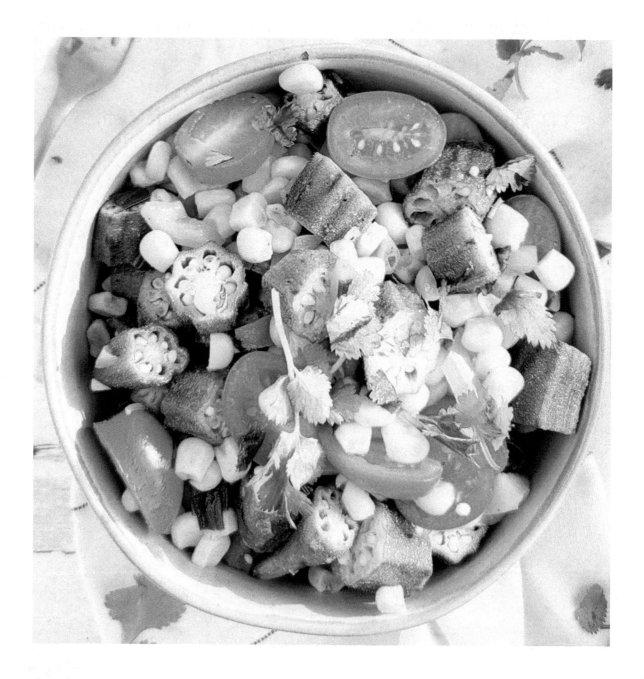

Preparation time: 10 minutes

Cooking time: 8 hours

Servings: 4

Ingredients:

- 3 garlic cloves, minced

- 1 small green bell pepper, chopped

- 1 small yellow onion, chopped

- 1 cup water

- 16 ounces okra, sliced

- 2 cups corn

- 1 and ½ teaspoon smoked paprika

- 28 ounces canned tomatoes, crushed

- 1 teaspoon oregano, dried

- 1 teaspoon thyme, dried

- 1 teaspoon marjoram, dried

- A pinch of cayenne pepper

- Salt and black pepper to the taste

Directions:

1. In your Slow cooker, mix garlic with bell pepper, onion, water, okra, corn, paprika, tomatoes, oregano, thyme, marjoram, cayenne, salt and pepper, cover, cook on Low for 8 hours, divide between plates and serve as a side dish.

Nutrition: calories 182, fat 3, fiber 6, carbs 8, protein 5

Mint Farro Pilaf

Preparation time: 10 minutes

Cooking time: 4 hours

Servings: 2

Ingredients:

- ½ tablespoon balsamic vinegar

- ½ cup whole grain farro

- A pinch of salt and black pepper

- 1 cup chicken stock

- ½ tablespoon olive oil

- 1 tablespoon green onions, chopped

- 1 tablespoon mint, chopped

Directions:

1. In your slow cooker, mix the farro with the vinegar and the other ingredients, toss, put the lid on and cook on Low for 4 hours.

2. Divide between plates and serve.

Nutrition: calories 162, fat 3, fiber 6, carbs 9, protein 4

Roasted Beets

Preparation time: 10 minutes

Cooking time: 4 hours

Servings: 5

Ingredients:

- 10 small beets

- 5 teaspoons olive oil

- A pinch of salt and black pepper

Directions:

1. Divide each beet on a tin foil piece, drizzle oil, season them with salt and pepper, rub well, wrap beets, place them in your Slow cooker, cover and cook on High for 4 hours.

2. Unwrap beets, cool them down a bit, peel, slice and serve them as a side dish.

Nutrition: calories 100, fat 2, fiber 2, carbs 4, protein 5

Parmesan Rice

Preparation time: 10 minutes

Cooking time: 2 hours and 30 minutes

Servings: 2

Ingredients:

- 1 cup rice

- 2 cups chicken stock

- 1 tablespoon olive oil

- 1 red onion, chopped

- 1 tablespoon lemon juice

- Salt and black pepper to the taste

- 1 tablespoon parmesan, grated

Directions:

1. In your slow cooker, mix the rice with the stock, oil and the other ingredients, toss, put the lid on and cook on High for 2 hours and 30 minutes.

2. Divide between plates and serve as a side dish.

Nutrition: calories 162, fat 4, fiber 6, carbs 29, protein 6

Thyme Beets

Preparation time: 10 minutes

Cooking time: 6 hours

Servings: 8

Ingredients:

- 12 small beets, peeled and sliced

- ¼ cup water

- 4 garlic cloves, minced

- 2 tablespoons olive oil

- 1 teaspoon thyme, dried

- Salt and black pepper to the taste

- 1 tablespoon fresh thyme, chopped

Directions:

1. In your Slow cooker, mix beets with water, garlic, oil, dried thyme, salt and pepper, cover and cook on Low for 6 hours.

2. Divide beets on plates, sprinkle fresh thyme all over and serve as a side dish.

Nutrition: 66, fat 4, fiber 1, carbs 8, protein 1

Spinach Rice

Preparation time: 10 minutes

Cooking time: 2 hours

Servings: 2

Ingredients:

- 2 scallions, chopped

- 1 tablespoon olive oil

- 1 cup Arborio rice

- 1 cup chicken stock

- 6 ounces spinach, chopped

- Salt and black pepper to the taste

- 2 ounces goat cheese, crumbled

Directions:

1. In your slow cooker, mix the rice with the stock and the other ingredients, toss, put the lid on and cook on High for 2 hours.

2. Divide between plates and serve as a side dish.

Nutrition: calories 300, fat 10, fiber 6, carbs 20, protein 14

Beets Side Salad

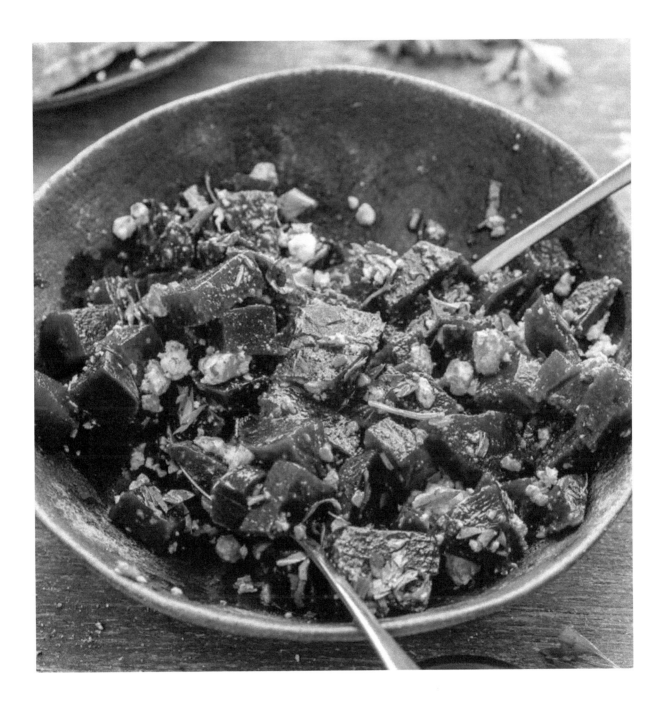

Preparation time: 10 minutes

Cooking time: 7 hours

Servings: 12

Ingredients:

- 5 beets, peeled and sliced

- ¼ cup balsamic vinegar

- 1/3 cup honey

- 1 tablespoon rosemary, chopped

- 2 tablespoons olive oil

- Salt and black pepper to the taste

- 2 garlic cloves, minced

Directions:

1. In your Slow cooker, mix beets with vinegar, honey, oil, salt, pepper, rosemary and garlic, cover and cook on Low for 7 hours.

2. Divide between plates and serve as a side dish.

Nutrition: calories 70, fat 3, fiber 2, carbs 17, protein 3

Mango Rice

Preparation time: 10 minutes

Cooking time: 2 hours

Servings: 2

Ingredients:

- 1 cup rice

- 2 cups chicken stock

- ½ cup mango, peeled and cubed

- Salt and black pepper to the taste

- 1 teaspoon olive oil

Directions:

1. In your slow cooker, mix the rice with the stock and the other ingredients, toss, put the lid on and cook on High for 2 hours.

2. Divide between plates and serve as a side dish.

Nutrition: calories 152, fat 4, fiber 5, carbs 18, protein 4

Lemony Beets

Preparation time: 10 minutes

Cooking time: 8 hours

Servings: 6

Ingredients:

- 6 beets, peeled and cut into medium wedges

- 2 tablespoons honey

- 2 tablespoons olive oil

- 2 tablespoons lemon juice

- Salt and black pepper to the taste

- 1 tablespoon white vinegar

- ½ teaspoon lemon peel, grated

Directions:

1. In your Slow cooker, mix beets with honey, oil, lemon juice, salt, pepper, vinegar and lemon peel, cover and cook on Low for 8 hours.

2. Divide between plates and serve as a side dish.

Nutrition: calories 80, fat 3, fiber 4, carbs 8, protein 4

Lemon Artichokes

Preparation time: 10 minutes

Cooking time: 3 hours

Servings: 2

Ingredients:

- 1 cup veggie stock

- 2 medium artichokes, trimmed

- 1 tablespoon lemon juice

- 1 tablespoon lemon zest, grated

- Salt to the taste

Directions:

1. In your slow cooker, mix the artichokes with the stock and the other ingredients, toss, put the lid on and cook on Low for 3 hours.

2. Divide artichokes between plates and serve as a side dish.

Nutrition: calories 100, fat 2, fiber 5, carbs 10, protein 4

Carrot and Beet Side Salad

Preparation time: 10 minutes

Cooking time: 7 hours

Servings: 6

Ingredients:

- ½ cup walnuts, chopped

- ¼ cup lemon juice

- ½ cup olive oil

- 1 shallot, chopped

- 1 teaspoon Dijon mustard

- 1 tablespoon brown sugar

- Salt and black pepper to the taste

- 2 beets, peeled and cut into wedges

- 2 carrots, peeled and sliced

- 1 cup parsley

- 5 ounces arugula

Directions:

1. In your Slow cooker, mix beets with carrots, salt, pepper, sugar, mustard, shallot, oil, lemon juice and walnuts, cover and cook on Low for 7 hours.

2. Transfer everything to a bowl, add parsley and arugula, toss, divide between plates and serve as a side dish.

Nutrition: calories 100, fat 3, fiber 3, carbs 7, protein 3

Coconut Bok Choy

Preparation time: 10 minutes

Cooking time: 1 hour

Servings: 2

Ingredients:

- 1 pound bok choy, torn

- ½ cup chicken stock

- ½ teaspoon chili powder

- 1 garlic clove, minced

- 1 teaspoon ginger, grated

- 1 tablespoon coconut oil

- Salt to the taste

Directions:

1. In your slow cooker, mix the bok choy with the stock and the other ingredients, toss, put the lid on and cook on High for 1 hour.

2. Divide between plates and serve as a side dish.

Nutrition: calories 100, fat 1, fiber 2, carbs 7, protein 4

Cauliflower and Carrot Gratin

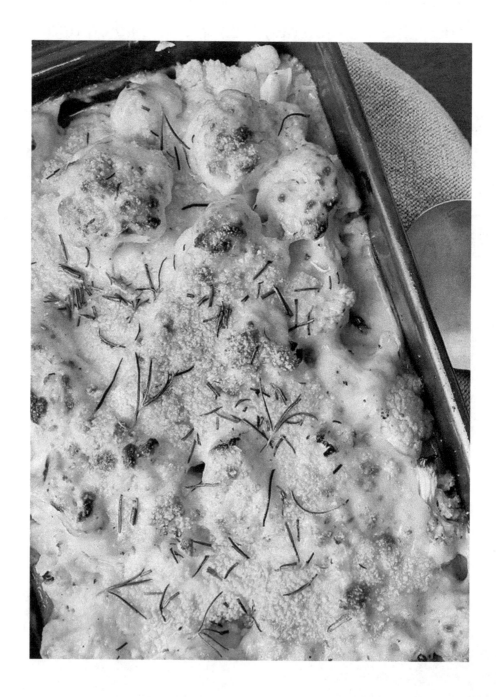

Preparation time: 10 minutes

Cooking time: 7 hours

Servings: 12

Ingredients:

- 16 ounces baby carrots

- 6 tablespoons butter, soft

- 1 cauliflower head, florets separated

- Salt and black pepper to the taste

- 1 yellow onion, chopped

- 1 teaspoon mustard powder

- 1 and ½ cups milk

- 6 ounces cheddar cheese, grated

- ½ cup breadcrumbs

Directions:

1. Put the butter in your Slow cooker, add carrots, cauliflower, onion, salt, pepper, mustard powder and milk and toss.

2. Sprinkle cheese and breadcrumbs all over, cover and cook on Low for 7 hours.

3. Divide between plates and serve as a side dish.

Nutrition: calories 182, fat 4, fiber 7, carbs 9, protein 4

Italian Eggplant

Preparation time: 10 minutes

Cooking time: 2 hours

Servings: 2

Ingredients:

- 2 small eggplants, roughly cubed

- ½ cup heavy cream

- Salt and black pepper to the taste

- 1 tablespoon olive oil

- A pinch of hot pepper flakes

- 2 tablespoons oregano, chopped

Directions:

1. In your slow cooker, mix the eggplants with the cream and the other ingredients, toss, put the lid on and cook on High for 2 hours.

2. Divide between plates and serve as a side dish.

Nutrition: calories 132, fat 4, fiber 6, carbs 12, protein 3

Conclusion

Did you take pleasure in trying these new and also delicious dishes? sadly we have come to the end of this vegetarian cookbook, I truly hope it has been to your taste. to enhance your wellness we want to encourage you to incorporate physical activity and a dynamic way of living in addition to adhere to these great recipes, so regarding emphasize the enhancements. we will be back soon with various other increasingly appealing vegan recipes, a huge hug, see you quickly.